Clinicians Update on the Treatment & Management of

Anxiety Disorders

DEBORAH ANTAI-OTONG

**For information on this and other PESI
manuals, audio recordings and seminars, please call
800-843-7763 or visit our website at www.pesi.com**

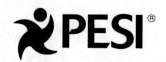

About the Author

Deborah Antai-Otong, MS, RN, PMH-NP, CS, is a certified specialist, educational, organizational and legal consultant. She is a national speaker on psychosocial topics including addiction, depression, anxiety disorders, dementia, psychopharmacology and psychiatric emergencies. Ms. Antai-Otong is also a motivational speaker on empowerment, caring for the caregiver, team building, anger management, conflict resolution and assertiveness training. She is the author of many publications including book chapters and journals, such as *American Journal of Nursing, Nursing, Nursing Clinics of North America, MED SURG Nursing, Geriatric Nursing* and *Journal of Addictions Nursing.* She is a member of several editorial and review boards including CLINICAL NURSE SPECIALIST, *Issues in Mental Health Nursing* and *Journal of Addictions Nursing.* Ms. Antai-Otong is also a manuscript reviewer for *Issues in Mental Health Nursing, Psychiatric Services* and psychosocial topics for *American Journal of Nursing.* She is the author of *Psychiatric Nursing: Biological and Behavioral Concepts* (W. B. Saunders) and co-author of *Decision-Making in Psychiatric and Psychosocial Nursing* (BC Decker, CV Mosby). Her clinical expertise includes psychiatric emergencies, medication management, crisis intervention and psychiatric consultation in clinical settings. Ms. Antai-Otong is also an expert communicator and organizational consultant helping staff improve work relationships through conflict resolution, anger management and team-building skills. She is a psychotherapist working with clients experiencing depression, grief, early childhood trauma and borderline personality disorders. She received her MS in psychiatric mental health nursing and BS from Texas Woman's University in Denton. She is also a Psychiatric Mental Health Nurse Practitioner.

Contents

Anxiety Disorders: An Overview

1

Introduction

Prevalence and Comorbidity of Anxiety Disorders

Anxiety disorders are serious medical conditions that affect roughly 19 million adults in America and they are ubiquitous across human cultures (Kessler, McGonagle, Zhao, et al, 1994; Weismman et al, 1997). They have a chronic, recurrent and relentless course. Research indicates that the lifetime prevalence of anxiety disorders is estimated to be as high as 25 percent and that about 1 in 4 people in the United States reports a lifetime history of at least 1 anxiety disorder (Kessler, McGonagle, Zhao, et al, 1994). Anxiety disorders are highly comorbid with each other and other mental health conditions especially mood disorders. These data also suggest that anxiety disorders carry a substantial burden of distress and suffering and disability comparable to chronic medical conditions, such as diabetes (Andrews, Sanderson & Beard, 1998; Kessler, Du Pont, Berglund & Wittchen, 1999). Economic cost of anxiety disorders include psychiatric and emergent care, hospitalization, prescription drugs, reduced productivity and suicide.

While they are treatable, less than a third of persons with anxiety disorders seek treatment (Lepine, 2002) Factors such as inaccurate diagnosis resulting in inappropriate treatment and chronicity also explain the high use of non-psychiatric services in persons presenting with anxiety disorders, particularly in primary care area (Greenberg, et al, 1999). Because individuals presenting with comorbid anxiety and other psychiatric conditions are often unrecognized, clinicians evaluate various anxiety disorders and implement appropriate interventions that reduce symptoms and promote an optimal level of functioning.

Causative Factors

There is growing evidence that indicates that anxiety disorder are multifaceted and arise from intricate neurochemical, neuroanatomical, genetic, and neuroendocrinologic factors. Cognitive-behavioral and environmental and stress influences also play a role in anxiety disorders (Antai-Otong, 2003).

Neurochemical theories point to dysregulation of several neurotransmitter, including excitatory, such as norepinephrine and serotonin and inhibitory, such as gamma amino-butyric acid (GABA) neurotransmitters as causative factors in anxiety disorders. Support of this theory is demonstrated in the efficacy of various pharmacological agents, such as benzodiazepine (e.g. clonazepam [Klonopin]) and antidepressants, including serotonin reuptake inhibitors (e.g. sertraline [Zoloft]).

Alterations in *neuroanatomical* structures including imprinting emotionally traumatic memories and conditioned fears that are mediated in the amygdala (encodes conditioned fear) through the hippocampus, which is involved in the storage and retrieval of fear-related memories and avoidance through the prefrontal cortex. The prefrontal lobe is involved in the assessment of likelihood of reward or punishment arising from past experiences. These structures are believed to play significant roles of the fear circuit by controlling mood shifts based on internal and external cues and modulating the stress response. Alterations in these regions give rise to exaggerated fear responses and avoidance behaviors that represent typical symptoms in various anxiety disorders, such as panic disorder, post traumatic stress disorder, generalized anxiety disorder and social phobia.

Genetic predisposition has been found in family and twin studies that indicate the heritability and predisposition of anxiety disorders.

Neuroendocrinologic studies implicate the hypothalamic pituitary adrenal (HPA) axis that effects cortisol secretion and modulation of the stress response. Examples of dysregulation of these processes are seen in individuals presenting with physical symptoms (e.g., increased heart rate, blood pressure, sweating, palpitations) of various anxiety disorders.

Cognitive-behavioral theorists submit that persons with anxiety disorders hold irrational and distorted beliefs about themselves, the world and the future. For instance, the person with GAD is often tense and worries extensively due to distorted beliefs about self (e.g. "I must be a bad parent because my adolescent flunked his math class.").

Clinical Features

Persons with anxiety disorders often present with an array of symptoms that range from exaggerated fear responses, such as post traumatic stress disorder (PTSD), to a need to perform ritualistic behaviors to reduce anxiety as seen in obsessive-compulsive disorder. Additional clinical features include "fear of fear" in persons with panic disorder. Clinical features of anxiety disorders provide the basis of integrated treatment models that reduce the intensity of physiological responses, alter cognitive and behavioral responses and promote a higher level of functioning and improve quality of life.

Summary

Despite the complexity of anxiety disorders, they are treatable. Because anxiety disorders often go unrecognized, it is imperative for clinicians to make differential diagnoses to distinguish normal anxiety from specific disorders and collaborate with the client, family and develop client-centered care that reduces the burden of anxiety disorders. This chapter is prelude to the following chapters that focus on specific anxiety disorders:

- Panic Disorder with and without a History of Agoraphobia
- Specific Phobia
- Social Phobia
- Obsessive-Compulsive Disorder (OCD)
- Posttraumatic Stress Disorder (PTSD)
- Generalized Anxiety Disorder (GAD)

Finally, this following chapters will also help clinicians identify symptoms of each anxiety disorder, understand their prevalence and course, causative factors, and effective treatment.

Suggested Reading

Andrews, G; Sanderson, K; & Beard, J (1998). Burden of disease: Methods of calculating disability from mental disorder. *British Journal of Psychiatry, 173,* 123–131.

Antai-Otong, D (2000). The neurobiology of anxiety disorders: Implications for psychiatric nursing practice, *Issues in Mental Health Nursing, 21,* 71–89.

Antai-Otong, D (2003). Anxiety disorders: Treatment considerations. *Nursing Clinics of North America, 38,* 35–44.

Greenberg, PE; Sisitsky, T; Kessler, RC; Finkelstein, SN; Berndt, ER; Davidson, JR; Ballenger, JC; & Fryer, AJ (1999). The economic burden of anxiety disorders in the 1990s. *Journal of Clinical Psychiatry, 60,* 427–435.

Kessler, RC; Du Pont, RL; Berglund, P; Wittchen, H-U (1999). Impairment in pure and comorbid generalized anxiety disorder and major depression at 12 months in two national surveys. *American Journal of Psychiatry, 156,* 1915–1923.

Kessler, RC; McGonagle, KA; Zhao, S; Nelson, CB; Hugnes, M; Eshleman, S; Wittchen, H-U; & Kendler, KS (1994). Lifetime and 12-month prevalence of DSM-III-R psychiatric disorders in the United States: Results from the National Comorbidity Survey. *Archives of General Psychiatry, 51:* 8–19.

Leon, AC; Portera, L; Weissman, MM (1995). The social costs of anxiety disorders. *British Journal of Psychiatry, 166* (suppl. 27): 19–22.

Lepine, JP (2002). The epidemiology of anxiety disorders: Prevalence and societal costs. *Journal of Clinical Psychiatry, 63,* Suppl. 14, 4–8.

Panic Disorders 2

Introduction

Persons with panic disorder have feeling of doom and terror that emerge suddenly, unexpectedly and repeatedly without warning. Common complaints also include palpitations, tingling sensations, nausea, chest discomfort, increased heart rate and blood pressure, sweating, dizziness and faintness. One-third of people with panic disorder also experience agoraphobia. People with panic disorder with agoraphobia are often fear-stricken and housebound. Because of their inability to predict when the next panic attack will occur, some clients resort to avoidance behaviors that can be disabling and impair their level of functioning. Despite these distressful symptoms, panic disorder is one of the most treatable anxiety disorders. This chapter focuses on panic disorder, its prevalence and treatment considerations.

Prevalence and Course

1. Panic disorder (PD) affects 2.4 million adults in this country and is twice as common in women as in men (Robins & Regier, 1990)
2. It affects 2% to 6% of the general population

3. The most common age of onset is between late adolescence, mid adulthood and rarely past the age of 50.

4. Clients with PD make frequent visits to the hospital emergency room or numerous medical visits before an accurate diagnosis is made.

5. PD is likely to be comorbid with other mental disorders, such as major depression, agoraphobia, alcoholism, social phobia, and PTSD.

6. Individuals with PD have a high rate of suicide.

7. Untreated PD can be extremely disabling and result in people becoming so restricted that they avoid normal and daily activities such as shopping or driving and in extreme cases becoming housebound due to fears of having another panic attack.

Causative Factors

1. Risk of developing PD appears to be genetic. First-degree biological relatives with this disorder are up to 8 times more likely to develop PD (American Psychiatric Association [APA], 2000; Hettema, Neale, & Kendler, 2001)

2. Dysregulation of several neurotransmitter systems are implicated in PD, namely norepinephrine, serotonin, and gamma amino-butyric acid (GABA)

3. Increased sympathetic nervous system tone that results in excessive responses to certain stimuli

4. Alterations in neuroanatomical regions of the brain (e.g., hippocampus)

Evaluation

Prior to treating the client who presents with an anxiety disorder an accurate diagnosis must be made. Making an accurate diagnosis requires establishing a therapeutic relationship with the client and performing a comprehensive evaluation that rules out psychiatric and medical conditions that mimic anxiety disorders. Once a definitive diagnosis is determined the clinician and client must collaborate and develop client-centered treatment. The following section focuses on strategies that assists clinicians in making a differential diagnosis of clients who present with panic disorder and other anxiety disorders.

Bio-Psychosocial Evaluation

1. Employ basic principles of caring for persons who present with psychiatric or mental conditions include

   a. Establish rapport

   b. Convey a caring, patient and empathetic attitude

2. Perform a bio-psychosocial evaluation that comprises:

   a. Identifying data

   b. Reasons for seeking treatment

   c. History of presenting symptoms with a focus on:

   - Onset, duration (usually discrete and episodic course) and their impact on the client's level of functioning
   - Questions about the course of symptoms—remitting or unremitting, precipitating events and associated disability, such as avoidance of large crowds, driving.
   - Questions about comorbid conditions, such as drug use, major depression (depression often accompanies PD and needs to be treated as well)

       • Physical, behavioral and emotional manifestations

  d. Current and past psychiatric treatment, including pre-scribed and over-the-counter medications/herbs, treatment adherence, and last appointment

  e. Present health status—including medications, past and present treatment

  f. Family history—psychiatric and medical conditions and treatment

  g. Quality of present support systems

  h. History of trauma or violence—as survivor or perpetrator, including domestic violence

3. Perform a Comprehensive Mental Status Examination

  a. General description of the client

  b. Appearance

  c. Mode of arrival

  d. Attitude towards clinician

  e. Eye contact (consider cultural factors)

  f. Psychomotor movements or behaviors (e.g., involuntary movements, pacing, tics, tremors)

  g. Behavior—level of activity

  h. Mood and Affect

  i. Characteristics of speech and language

  j. Perceptions

  k. Thought Processes

  l. Thought Content

  m. Concentration and attention

  n. Sensorium and cognition

  o. Orientation

p. Ability to abstract

q. Memory—recent, remote, and immediate recall

r. Judgement

s. Insight

t. Reliability

4. Determine the Client's Level of Dangerousness to Self and Others (Suicide and Homicide Assessment)

   a. Risk Factors

   - Factors that increase the risk of suicide in the anxious client include comorbid psychiatric and substance-related disorders such as major depression and alcoholism; a sense of helplessness and powerlessness that often underscore avoidance behaviors and a overwhelming loss of control over symptoms unique to specific anxiety disorders.

   b. Additional risk factors

   - Previous history of attempts
   - Family history of suicide
   - Significant losses
   - Demographics (e.g. older white males)
   - Comorbid psychiatric conditions
   - A sense of hopelessness
   - Lack of quality support system
   - Ineffective coping skills

Clear and concise documentation of findings from this evaluation is imperative for all clients presenting with anxiety and other psychiatric disorders. This data must be legibly written and is important for clinical and legal purposes.

Differential Medical Diagnoses

Clients presenting with acute symptoms of anxiety require a basic medical evaluation that facilitates making differential diagnoses. Studies indicate that the client with psychiatric symptoms is likely to have comorbid medical conditions, cognitive disturbances and substance-related disorders. Clinicians working with anxious clients have a propensity to overlook medical conditions that mimic anxiety disorders. Accurately diagnosing presenting symptoms is crucial to working with the client and developing and implementing an appropriate treatment plan. A basic template of the evaluation process for clients that present with symptoms of anxiety follows:

1. Current vital signs—abnormal findings may indicate underlying medical, neurologic, or medication-induced conditions

2. Physical observations—review of symptoms, medications and substance misuse

3. Results of last physical examination

4. Basic laboratory and diagnostic screens

- Complete blood count with differential
- Chemistry panel
- Urinalysis
- Toxicology screens, including blood alcohol levels (BAL)
- Liver panel
- Renal studies
- Cardiovascular status—electrocardiogram (ECG)
- Pregnancy in test (child bearing age group)
- Thyroid panel
- Tests for sexually transmitted diseases when appropriate
- Vitamin B_{12}, folate, and thiamine levels—especially in older adults and clients with a history of chronic alcoholism

In brief, data gathered from the psychosocial assessment and physical screening serves as the basis of medical or psychiatric diagnosis and guide clinicians in the treatment planning process. A medical diagnosis requires an immediate referral for a comprehensive physical evaluation and treatment.

Typical Presentation of Client with Panic Disorder

Symptoms have a sudden and discreet onset of apprehension, fearfulness or terror associated with feelings of doom followed by at least one month of persistent concern about having another attack. (*See* **Table I**)

Physical Findings

Sudden and discreet onset of apprehension, fearfulness, or terror associated with feelings of doom and accompanied by:

- Dizziness and lightheadedness
- Shortness of breath (SOB)
- Diaphoresis (sweating)
- Parethesias (numbness and tingling sensations)
- Tachycardia (increased heart rate)
- Increased respirations
- Upset stomach, including diarrhea
- Muscle tension
- Restlessness
- Palpitations
- Trembling and Shakiness
- Chest pain or discomfort

Mental Status Examination

- Derealization
- Depersonalization
- Concentration and attention disturbances
- Intense fears
- Avoidant behaviors
- Persistent concerns about having additional attacks
- Fears of losing control, "going crazy, dying or having a heart attack"
- Fear of open spaces/places (e.g., shopping, driving) or situations in which escape is difficult or embarrassing, and housebound*

(APA, 2000)

Table I: Major Symptoms of Panic Disorder

Client must experience:

- Recurrent or unexpected panic attacks for at least 1 month or longer following the attack:
- Severe anxiety or concern about having additional attacks
- Significant change in behavior due to the attacks
- Attacks are not due to the direct physiological effects of a general medical condition or substance
- Attacks are not better accounted for by another psychiatric or mental condition

(APA, 2000)

Treatment Considerations

Once a definitive diagnosis of PD is made, clinicians must collaborate with the client and family to determine a course of treatment. Families

---

* With agoraphobia

play a crucial role in the treatment of anxiety disorders and clinicians need to provide health education about PD and available treatment options. They must also be allowed to discuss their feelings and concerns about the client's condition.

Pharmacological Interventions

There is mounting evidence that indicates that an integrated model that includes pharmacological and non-pharmacological interventions are likely to yield better treatment outcomes for clients with PD (APA, 1998). The first-line treatment of PD involves an integrated model of care that combines pharmacological interventions using antidepressants such as selective serotonin reuptake inhibitors (SSRIs), novel agents, benzodiazepines and cognitive behavioral therapy (CBT). The efficacy of pharmacological intervention lies in their ability to correct underlying neurobiological processes that contribute to physiological aspects of PD. (*See* **Table II:** Common Medications used in the Treatment of Panic Disorder). (*See* **Appendix A:** Major Side Effects Associated with SSRIs)

Cognitive-Behavioral Therapy and Other Psychosocial Interventions

The usefulness of CBT and other non-pharmacological interventions lies in teaching clients how to view panic attacks differently by learning how to challenge underlying distorted or false beliefs about mild somatic (physical) sensations and eliminate beliefs and behaviors that maintain PD symptoms. CBT and other psychotherapies require advanced education and training. The cognitive component of CBT further teaches the client that when attacks do occur they are short-lived and non-life threatening. For example, a client complaining of dying during a panic attack can be taught that these attacks are not life-threatening and that they can control symptoms with medications

Table II: Common Medications Used in the Treatment of Panic Disorder			
SSRIs	Other Antidepressants	Benzodiazepines	Beta Blockers
Fluoxetine (Prozac) Sertraline (Zoloft)* Escitalopram (Lexapro) Citalopram (Celexa) Paroxetine (Paxil)*	Monamine oxidase inhibitor (MAOI) Phenelzine (Nardil) Tricyclic anti- depressants Imipramine (Tofranil)	Clonazepam (Klonopin) Alprazaolam* and Extended Release (X-R) (Xanax) Lorazepam (Ativan)	Propanolol (Inderal)

* FDA approved for the treatment of PD

and/or deep breathing exercises. The behavioral component of CBT helps the client modify his/her reaction to anxiety-provoking situations, such as driving a car. Generally, CBT training lasts about 12 weeks and may involve an individual or group approach

Deep abdominal breathing exercises, stress management and other relaxation techniques are also useful in reducing the intensity of panic attacks and physiological manifestations of PD and enhancing the effects of treatment. Avoidance of known drugs that induce anxiety, such as caffeine, over-the-counter drugs cold preparation (e.g. pseudoephedrine) or illicit drugs (e.g., methamphetamine, cocaine) can also precipitate symptoms of anxiety.

Summary

Panic disorder has lifetime prevalence between 1% to 3%. Its high comorbidity with major depression and alcoholism challenges clinicians to recognize symptoms and make an accurate diagnosis to afford timely and appropriate treatment. This chapter has focused on salient treatment issues for the client presenting with panic disorder. As more and more research explores the efficacy of pharmacological agents and other treatment approaches, clients will have even greater opportunities to manage their symptoms, improve their quality of life and reduce the disabling effects of PD.

Suggested Reading

American Psychiatric Association (1998). Practice guideline for the treatment of patients with panic disorder. *American Journal of Psychiatry, 155* (5 Suppl.), 1–34.

American Psychiatric Association (2000). *Diagnostic and statistical manual of mental disorders, 4th edition, Text Revision.* Washington, DC.

Antai-Otong, D (2003). Anxiety disorders: Treatment considerations. *Nursing Clinics of North America, 38,* 35–44.

Beck, AT; Emery, G; & Greenberg, R (1985). *Anxiety disorders and phobias: A cognitive perspective.* New York: Basic Books.

Hettema, JM; Neale, MC; & Kendler, KS (2001). A review and meta-analysis of the genetic epidemiology of anxiety disorders. *American Journal of Psychiatry, 158,* 1568–1578.

Otto, MW; Tuby, KS; Gould, RA; McLean, RY; & Pollack, MH (2001). An effect-size analysis of the relative efficacy and tolerability of serotonin reuptake inhibitors for panic disorder. *American Journal of Psychiatry, 158,* 1989–1992.

Robins, LN & Regier, DA (1991). *Psychiatric disorders in America: The Epidemiologic Catchment Area Study.* New York: The Free Press.

Phobias 3

Introduction

Phobias

Persons with phobias often present with complaints of marked fear of a specific object or situation. They also report that exposure to these fear-provoking conditions elicit intense anxiety that include full-blown panic attacks or avoidance behaviors. Most people with phobias realize that their fears are irrational and unreasonable, such as a fear of heights, spiders, flying and earthquakes. While most may not experience debilitating effects from their fears, others may be paralyzed by theirs and require treatment. This chapter focuses on major phobias, such as specific phobias and social phobia or social anxiety. More attention will center on the later anxiety disorder because of its tendency to produce marked, persistent and disabling anxiety associated with significant and prolonged anticipatory anxiety that interferes with social performance and overall functioning.

Specific Phobias

Prevalence and Course

1. While phobias are common in the general population, they are unlikely to produce distress or disability that necessitate a diagnosis of Specific Phobia.

2. Current studies indicate that an estimated 8 percent of the adult population experiences one or more specific phobias in one year (American Psychiatric Association [APA], 2000)

3. Normally, the course of specific phobias emerges during childhood and may peak during the mid-20s.

4. Regardless of when they begin, most phobias endure for years or even decades with relatively limited remission without treatment.

Unlike other phobias, specific phobias do not result from exposure to a single traumatic incident, such as being bitten by a snake. Instead, there is data that suggest that phobia in family members and social or vicarious learning of phobias is the basis of these disorders. Typically, the client with a specific phobia focuses on a fear or avoidance such as animal type (e.g., dog, insects); natural environment type (e.g., earthquake, tornado) or situational type (e.g., elevator, tunnel). The most common type is situational and the least is the animal type (APA, 2000). Adults with these disorders recognize that their fears are exaggerated or unreasonable. Treatment of these disorders varies and depends upon the intensity and degree of impairment. If the level of distress does not produce significant distress or impairment, a diagnosis is not made. In contrast, if the client experiences marked and persistent fear cued by the presence or anticipation of a specific situation or object and/or precipitates a panic attack and avoidance behavior, a diagnosis may be warranted (APA, 2000). Differential diagnosis that rules out other psychiatric or medical conditions must also be made prior to making this diagnosis.

Because most clients with specific phobias are unlikely to seek treatment or experience disabling symptoms, an in-depth discussion of this disorder is unnecessary. Instead, the remainder of this chapter will focus primarily on social phobia because of its high morbidity and the likelihood of clients to seek treatment.

Social Phobia

Introduction

Social phobia, also referred to as social anxiety, is characterized by overwhelming anxiety and extreme self-consciousness in normal everyday social interactions. Major fears of persons concern the possibility of embarrassment, humiliation and ridicule. They often report histories of preoccupation with concerns that others will see their anxiety symptoms—sweaty palms, shaky voice or notice their hesitant and rapid speech and judge them as "stupid, inept or weak." Persons with social phobia are also likely to report having intense anticipatory anxiety for days or weeks prior to the "dreaded" event.

Prevalence and Course

1. According to data from the National Comorbidity Survey social phobia (social anxiety disorder) has a lifetime prevalence of 13.3 percent (Kessler, et al, 1994) These data indicate that an estimated 5.3 million people in this country have social phobia in any given year.

2. Women are twice as likely than men to suffer from social phobia

3. Normally, social phobia begins during childhood or early adolescence and seldom develops after the age of 25.

4. The onset of symptoms often follow an embarrassing or humiliating experience or it may be subtle

5. Comorbid psychiatric conditions are prevalent in persons with social phobia

6. Generally, most people with social phobia fear public speaking, using public bathrooms or eating in public places

Causative Factors

Similar to other anxiety disorders, causes of social phobia are multifaceted and include:

1. A familial pattern, especially the generalized subtype. *Generalized type* refers to intense anxiety and fears that occurs anytime the person is around others. In contrast to persons who only experience one specific type or situation, such as public speaking, the generalized type is likely to be more severe and very debilitating (APA, 2000).

2. Recent studies also implicate alterations in the amygdala that contribute to the intense fear responses associated with social phobia and dysregulation of neuroendocrine structures (e.g., hippocampus [HPA]) that may explain the heightened sensitivity to disapproval

3. Environmental factors associated with observational learning and social modeling may also play a role in social phobia

Evaluation

A general description of the evaluation process has been previously discussed in Chapter 2. In addition to establishing a therapeutic relationship, performing a comprehensive bio-psychosocial evaluation and medical screening, clinicians must rule out medical and psychiatric conditions. Oftentimes, clients with social phobia fail to report a full perspective about their social fears so it is imperative for clinicians to review a list of social and performance situation. Questions, such as "Describe what its like for you to do a presentation at a staff meeting" can provide clearer picture of the client's distress. Because of the high comorbidity of psychiatric disorders, such as alcoholism and major depression, a differential diagnosis is crucial to the treatment planning of clients with social phobia. The following data may be gathered when evaluating a client with social phobia:

Physical Findings

- Blushing
- Stomach or abdominal distress (e.g., nausea)
- Diaphoresis (sweating)
- Trembling and shakiness
- Difficulty speaking
- Poor interpersonal skills manifested by poor eye contact (consider cultural factors)
- Cold clammy and sweaty hands
- Fatigue

Mental Status Examination

- Shyness
- Heightened fear of disapproval, rejection and criticism
- Low self-esteem
- Excessive fear of being around others or situations
- Low and hesitant voice
- Feelings of inferiority
- Depressed or sad mood

- Suicidal ideations
- Concentration disturbances

Table III: Major Symptoms of Social Anxiety Disorder

- Marked and intense fear of one or more social performance situations involving unfamiliar people or possibly criticism by other
- Exposure to the feared social situation that normally generates intense anxiety
- The person recognizes that the fear is unreasonable and exaggerated
- Avoidance of the situation
- Avoidance behavior impairs functioning
- If under the age of 18, the duration is at least 6 months
- Not due to a substance or general medical condition

APA (2000)

When an accurate diagnosis is made, the clinician must work with the client and family members and develop a treatment plan that involves reducing the distress of specific fears, increase self-esteem and promote a sense of control and mastery of symptoms and life.

Treatment Considerations

Contemporary studies indicate that there are two effective forms of treatment available to clients with social phobia (Liebowitz, Heimberg, Schneier, Hope, Davies, et al, 1999). Researchers further contend that the long-term effects of CBT are superior to phenelzine (Nardil), a MAOI. These data strengthen debate concerning the efficacy of an integrated model of care in the treatment of social anxiety disorder and other anxiety disorders. These interventions are similar to those previously discussed in Chapter 2 and include pharmacological and short-term psychotherapy that integrates cognitive behavioral therapy (CBT) and other psychosocial interventions such as relaxation techniques and deep abdominal breathing exercises.

Pharmacological Interventions

Similar to the treatment of PD, medications that have proven efficacy in the treatment of social phobia include SSRIs, MAOIs, high-potency benzodiazepines and beta-blockers, such as propanol (Inderal). Clients must be cautioned about abrupt discontinuation of any medications, but particularly benzodiazepines. Abrupt discontinuation of antidepressants may precipitate an anticholinergic rebound or discontinuation syndrome. Of greater concern is the risk of withdrawal seizures when benzodiazepines are abruptly withdrawn.

Cognitive-Behavioral Therapy and Other Psychosocial Interventions

The efficacy of CBT lies in its ability to teach the client how to modify his/her perception of frightening situations. Exposure therapy is one such approach. Normally, exposure therapy consists of three steps. The first step involves introducing the client to the feared situation. This must follow a discussion about the aim of exposure therapy and its benefits. The client must be prepared and agreeable to the approach. During the second step, clients are encouraged to visualize situations that evoke their fears and perceived criticism. The third step entails educating the client about techniques that strengthen coping skills and mastery of disapproval. Relaxation techniques that include deep abdominal breathing exercises are also useful in anxiety management to manage varying levels of anxiety and enhance other treatment strategies.

Summary

Social phobia or social anxiety disorder is one of the most prevalent anxiety disorders. It has the potential to impact clients in specific social situations or in every social interaction. The potential disabling impact of this disorder requires astute clinical skills that enable clients to be treated in a timely and appropriate manner. This chapter has focused on major treatment considerations that offer hope and guidance in the treatment of social phobia.

Suggested Reading

American Psychiatric Association (2000). *Diagnostic and statistical manual of mental disorders, 4th edition, Text Revision.* Washington, DC.

Antai-Otong, D (2003). Anxiety disorders: Treatment considerations. *Nursing Clinics of North America, 38,* 35–44.

Beck, AT; Emery, G; & Greenberg, R (1985). *Anxiety disorders and phobias: A cognitive perspective.* New York: Basic Books.

Liebowitz; MR; Heimberg, RG; Schneier, FR; Hope, DA; Davies, S; Holt, CS; Goetz, D; Juster, HR; Lin, SH; Bruch, MA; Marshall, RD; Klein, DF (1999). Cognitive-behavioral group therapy versus phenelzine in social phobia: long-term outcome. *Depress Anxiety, 10,* 89–98.

National Institute of Mental Health (NIMH) website for information about social phobia and other anxiety disorders:
http://www.nimh.nih.gov/anxiety/anxiety.cfm

Obsessive-Compulsive Disorder

4

Introduction

Persons with obsessive-compulsive disorder (OCD) complain about obsessions and compulsions. *Obsessions* are recurrent, intrusive, and distressful ideas, impulses or images that are perceived as unreasonable, irrational, pointless, uncontrollable and forbidden. Common obsessive themes include contamination with germs, doubts, order or symmetry. Images or impulses generate marked significant personal distress anxiety and is normally relieved by compulsions or rituals aimed at relieving distress or preventing specific foreboding events. *Compulsions* are repetitive behaviors such as hand washing, showering or mental acts (e.g., praying, counting, and walking on certain floor or ground patterns). Sometimes these rituals consume a great deal of the client's time and may produce damaging results, such as skin excoriation from too much washing or showering. Unfortunately, these rituals offer the client temporary relief from disturbing thoughts or images that increase when they are not performed. (American Psychiatric Association [APA], 2000)

Prevalence and Course

1. Most data demonstrate a lifetime prevalence of OCD between 0.5 percent to 2.1 percent in adults and 1 percent to 2.3 percent in children and adolescents

2. OCD affects 3.3 million adults in this country (Robins & Regier, 1991)

3. OCD occurs equally in men and women

4. The onset of OCD may begin in childhood, but it usually begins in adolescence or early adulthood. Normally the onset is earlier in males than females, between the age of 6 to 15 years in males and 20 years to 29 years in females (APA, 2000).

5. The course is often insidious, with acute onsets in some cases.

6. Most persons experience a fluctuating course that may be generated by environmental stress

7. Common comorbidities include major depression, other anxiety disorders, substance-related disorders and eating disorders (Regier, Rae, Narrow, et al, 1998)

8. Fifteen percent of persons with OCD experience a deteriorating course that results in impaired occupational and social functioning

9. One-third of adults with OCD experienced their initial symptoms as children

Causative Factors

1. OCD, has a stronger familial pattern or genetic predisposition than most other anxiety disorders

2. There is also an increased vulnerability of OCD among first-degree relatives with Tourette's syndrome

3. Fifty percent of persons with Tourette's disorder develop OCD

4. OCD behaviors is also found in persons with body dysmorphic disorder because of preoccupation with one's appearance

5. Dysregulation in various neurotransmitter systems including serotonergic and dopaminergic systems

6. Alterations in neuroanatomical structures associated with increased activity in the frontal lobes and basal ganglia

7. National Institute of Mental Health (NIMH) studies of OCD in young people have demonstrated that having group A streptococcus bacterial infection may result in the development of disabling obsessions and compulsions. Vulnerability to this the streptococcal form of OCD is associated with a genetics or familial pattern and rheumatic fever. Initial research indicates that distinct treatment for the infection improves or alleviates the OCD.

Evaluation

Basic principles associated with establishing rapport and a therapeutic relationship are the crucial to evaluating clients present with OCD. A discussion of the evaluation process is discussed in Chapter 2 and includes the bio-psychosocial evaluation, physical screening and mental status examination. When screening children or young people a history of infections must be part of the evaluation to rule out streptococcal-induced OCD. This differential diagnosis is crucial to the client receiving appropriate treatment for the infection. The following discussion explicates common findings in clients with OCD:

Physical Findings

- Skin or dermatological conditions resulting from excessive water or caustic cleaning agents
- Extremely dry or chapped hands
- Fatigue

Mental Status Examination

- Preoccupation with obsessions and compulsions
- Insight that their behavior is pointless and irrational
- Children may lack insight into their behavior
- Expressed need to wash hands after a handshake or touching objects
- Avoidance of activities perceived to be associated with contamination or other obsessional themes
- Pathological doubt followed by the need to count or check
- Sad or depressed mood
- Exaggerated guilt
- Suicidal ideations/gestures
- Concentration or attention disturbances

Table IV: Major Symptoms of OCD

Either Obsessions or Compulsions

Obsessions

- Recurrent and persistent thoughts, ideas, images that are irrational, intrusive and inappropriate and result in significant anxiety and personal distress
- Person attempts to eliminate or neutralize thoughts, ideas, or images with other activities
- Person recognizes that obsessions are pointless, irrational

<u>Compulsions</u>

- Repetitive behaviors used to eliminate or neutralize obsessions and the person feels driven to perform these rituals

The obsessions and compulsions produce profound distress and impairment. The disturbances are not related to a substance or general medical condition.

(APA, 2000)

Treatment Considerations

Effective treatment for OCD is similar to other anxiety disorders and includes an integrated model that combines pharmacological and psychosocial interventions. The client and clinician must collaborate and discern the best treatment strategies.

Pharmacological Interventions

Antidepressants have demonstrated high efficacy in the treatment of OCD because they provide a broad-spectrum of activity with proven efficacy in the treatment of this disorder and comorbid depression. The first medication specifically approved for the use in the treatment of OCD was the tricyclic antidepressant (TCA) clomipramine (Anafranil). Additional drugs that have proven efficacy in the treatment of OCD are the SSRIs, fluvoxamine (Luvox), fluoxetine (Prozac), paroxetine (Paxil) and sertraline (Zoloft). Health education about the use of pharmacologic agents; withdrawal symptoms and side effects to report must be an integral part of medication management in the treatment of OCD.

Cognitive-Behavioral Therapy and Other Psychosocial Interventions

The efficacy of CBT in the treatment of anxiety disorders, including OCD, is well documented. The behavioral component of CBT is especially effective in the treatment of OCD, namely exposure and response prevention. The usefulness of exposure and response prevention can be demonstrated in helping the client who fears germs confront the discomfort by asking the client to touch a doorknob. This enables the client to go a designated period without washing and cope with resultant anxiety. Ultimately, after this exercise has been repeated several times, anxiety will abate. This exercise must be individually tailored to meet the client's unique concerns and implemented when the client is ready.

Summary

OCD is a complex anxiety disorder that stems from diverse causative factors. Clinicians are challenged to make an accurate diagnosis that guides treatment planning. Helping the client understand reasons for obsessions and compulsions is challenging, but is crucial to successful resolution or management of these distressful symptoms. As with other anxiety disorders, it is imperative for the clinician to collaborate with the client in developing an individualized plan of care that improves self-esteem, confidence, restores control over one's life and promotes a higher level of functioning.

Suggested Reading

American Psychiatric Association (2000). *Diagnostic and statistical manual of mental disorders, 4th edition, Text Revision.* Washington, DC.

Beck, AT; Emery, G; & Greenberg, R (1985). *Anxiety disorders and phobias: A cognitive perspective.* New York: Basic Books.

Regier, DA; Rae, DS; Narrow, WE; Kaebler, CT; & Schatzberg, AF (1998). Prevalence of anxiety disorders and their comorbidity with mood and addictive disorders. *British Journal of Psychiatry Supplement, 34,* 24–28.

Robins, LN & Regier, DA (1990). *Psychiatric disorders in America: The Epidemiologic Catchment Area Study.* New York: The Free Press.

Post-Traumatic Stress Disorder

5

Introduction

Post-traumatic stress disorder (PTSD) is an anxiety disorder that can result from exposure to an overwhelming or traumatic experience in which grave harm occurred or was threatened. Traumatic or severely stressful experiences that can precede the development of PTSD include those that threatened physical integrity—rape, witnessing a murder, natural or human-related disasters, accidents, or military combat. Clients often present with complaints of intrusive thoughts or memories of the event, flashbacks, nightmares hyperarousal, hyper-vigilant and avoidance behaviors (American Psychiatric Association [APA], 2000).

Prevalence and Course

1. Approximately 3.6 percent of U.S. adults ages 18 to 54 or 5.2 million people have PTSD during the course of a given year. Of whom about 30 percent of men and women symptoms follow time spend in war zones. One million war veterans developed PTSD following their tours in Vietnam. Estimates up to

8 percent of PTSD have been found in veterans of the Persian Gulf War. The Iraqi War is likely to produce an undetermined number of veterans with PTSD (NIMH PTSD Facts).

2. Rates of PTSD in child and adult survivors of violence and disaster range from 2 percent after a natural disaster to 29 percent following a plane crash

3. Women are more likely than men to develop PTSD

4. Susceptibility (across the life span) may run in families

5. Comorbid conditions associated with PTSD include depression, substance-related and other anxiety disorders, such as panic disorder.

6. Not everyone who is exposed to a traumatic or overwhelming stressful encounter develops PTSD

7. PTSD is only diagnosed if symptoms persist longer than 1 month

8. Symptoms usually emerge within 3 months of the trauma and the course varies: some people recover within 6 months, while other symptoms persist much longer (chronic)

Causative Factors

1. Findings from animal studies indicate that early stress is associated with alterations in the hippocampus and may be associated with chronic PTSD (e.g., shrinkage in volume) (a brain region that plays a crucial role in learning and memory)

2. Studies of animals and humans have pinpointed the specific brain regions and circuits involved in anxiety and fear, which are significant in understanding PTSD and other anxiety disorders. It has been found that the fear response is mediated by a small structure in the brain, called the amygdala, that is

believed to be associated with abnormal or exaggerated activation of the fear response in persons with PTSD.

3. Alterations (high levels) in the stress hormones (e.g., cortisol and endorphins) that temporarily mask pain and account for "numbing" or blunted emotions in persons with PTSD

4. Childhood sexual abuse is a significant public health problem that affects 16 percent of women in America a at some time prior to their 18th birthday (McCauley, et al, 1997) and is a frequent cause of PTSD (Saigh & Bremner, 1999)

5. Factors that influence the risk of PTSD include:

   - Characteristics of the trauma (proximity and duration)
   - Characteristics of the person (e.g. previous trauma, psychiatric illness [personal and family])
   - Gender—women are at the greatest risk for traumatic experiences
   - Post trauma factors (e.g., quality of support systems, emergence of avoidance/numbing, hyperarousal, or intrusive or recurring memories

Evaluation

A thorough and comprehensive mental status examination that includes queries about past trauma and recent trauma and physical screening are crucial to making a diagnosis of PTSD. The evaluation also involves assessing the severity of trauma, including type, duration and proximity. Efforts to rule out other psychiatric conditions such as major depression, substance abuse and other anxiety disorders must be a part of the differential diagnosis. Because PTSD symptoms are similar to *acute stress disorder* (ASD), it is imperative for clinicians to assess the time of the trauma and severity of symptoms. A primary distinction between ASD and PTSD is duration of symptoms. ASD symptoms follow exposure to a traumatic or overwhelming stressful situation, and occur within 4 weeks of the event and resolve within this period. In contrast PTSD symptoms last more than a month.

The following clinical findings are common in people presenting with PTSD:

Physical Findings (Adults)

- Increased heart rate and blood pressure
- Hyperarousal (exaggerated startle response)—sensitive to sounds, movements, close proximity
- Diaphoresis
- Sleep disturbances associated with nightmares and flashbacks
- Fatigue
- Depressed or sad mood
- Tearfulness
- Agitation
- Irritability

Mental Status Examination (Adults)

- Concentration disturbances, possibly related to recurrent or intrusive thoughts/memories
- Avoidance behaviors
- Depersonalization
- Survivor's guilt
- Suicidal or homicidal ideations
- Derealization
- Significant anxiety
- Restricted affect
- Marked loss of interest in things that were once pleasurable

- Isolation or distancing from others
- Hypervigilance
- Suspiciousness or distrust
- Flashbacks
- Feelings of helplessness and powerlessness
- Fear or panic

Physical Findings (Children)

- Sleep disturbances
- Complain of stomachaches
- Fatigues

Mental Status (Children)

- Depressed and sad mood
- Irritable mood
- Anxiety
- Acting out behavior at home or school
- Decline in academic performance
- Emotional numbness or flatness
- Regressive behaviors
- Nightmares

Table VI: Major Symptoms of Post-traumatic Stress Disorder

A. Exposure to a traumatic or overwhelming stressful and life threatening situation/event that generates intense fear, marked anxiety and horror
   In children it may be expressed in disorganized agitation

B. The traumatic event/encounter is persistently relived or re-experienced in one or more of the following:

- Intrusive thoughts, memories or images of the event
- Recurrent nightmares or dreams
- Reliving the event (flashbacks, illusions)
- Marked psychological distress at exposure to internal or external cues that represent the trauma

Biological reactivity on exposure to internal or external cues that depict the trauma

C. Prolonged avoidance of the stimuli linked to the trauma and emotional numbing as manifested by:

- Avoid places, people or things
- Difficulty recalling an important part of the trauma
- Significant loss of interest or participation in important daily activities
- Feelings of detachment or alienation from others
- Restricted affect
- Sense of a foreboding future

D. Prolonged symptoms of hyperarousal as evidenced by:

- Sleep disturbances
- Irritable mood and outbursts of anger
- Concentration disturbances
- Hypervigilance
- Exaggerated startle response
- Symptoms persist longer than 1 month
- Disturbance produces profound distress and impairs overall functioning

(APA, 2000)

Treatment Considerations

PTSD is a potentially disabling anxiety disorder. After making a diagnosis, clinicians must work with the client and develop a treatment plan that facilitates healthy resolution of the trauma. Some studies indicate that offering an opportunity to talk about their experiences very soon after a traumatic experience may reduce the severity of PTSD symptoms. Clinicians must afford adequate time for the evaluation and promote a safe environment that facilitates discussion of the trauma. This process requires patience on the part of the clinician and client. Treatment must be integrated and target both the physiological manifestations of PTSD along with the cognitive aspects. Understandably, treatment for PTSD consists of medications and cognitive behavioral therapy and other psychosocial interventions.

Pharmacological Interventions

There is no simple rule that determines the choice of pharmacological interventions for clients presenting with PTSD. Major drugs that have proven efficacy in the treatment of PTSD are the SSRIs (e.g., sertraline [Zoloft], paroxetine [Paxil], citalopram [Celexa]), particularly during the early stage of this disorder. Clearly, SSRIs are the first-line treatment for PTSD. Their efficacy lies in their broad-spectrum properties to reduce the severity all three PTSD symptom clusters and manage comorbid conditions, such as depression and other anxiety disorders. These agents also have a low side effect profile and enhance the client's overall level of functioning. Another agent with proven efficacy, especially in the management of exaggerated physical responses (e.g., hyperarousal) is propranolol (Inderal). When given shortly after the acute traumatization propranol significantly reduced physiological reactivity to trauma cues or stimuli (Pitman, Sanders, Zusman, et al, 2002). Researchers continue to search for the ideal pharmacological agents for the treatment of PTSD.

Cognitive-Behavioral Therapy and Other Psychosocial Interventions

One of the most proven forms of cognitive behavioral therapies for of PTSD is exposure therapy. The premise behind the efficacy of exposure therapy is based on the notion that PTSD represents an exaggerated or pathological fear circuitry in memory, which is thought to depict stimuli, responses and their meaning. The memory structure is activated by trauma-related data (e.g., internal or external cues). Persons with PTSD are believed to have a large number of stimuli and response representations in their trauma fear circuitry that is easily accessed and result in PTSD symptoms.

Exposure therapy consists of several approaches: systematic desensitization (imaginal or vivo), implosive therapy, flooding, self-control desensitization and other techniques. Imaginal exposure typically involves repeated reliving of the traumatic encounter. The goal of exposure therapy is emotional reprocessing that involves correcting the exaggerated or pathological fear circuitry.

Prior to initiating exposure therapy, the client must agree to participate. Normally, this occurs when the client feels safe. A supportive and safe environment is crucial to the success of exposure therapy. In general, the clinician confronts or exposes the client to trauma-related data and activates the trauma memory, which enables the client to modify or correct data to be integrated in the trauma memory and alter the pathological elements of the memory. Repetitive exposure or reliving the trauma facilitates successful resolution of the trauma (Rothbaum & Foa, 1999). This specialized form of CBT, like other psychotherapies, requires advanced educational preparation and clinical expertise, especially in the area of child and adolescent trauma cases.

A newer form of exposure therapy is Virtual Reality Exposure (VRE) in which the client is presented with a computer generated view of a virtual world that changes with head motion. During these sessions, clients clad the head-mounted display with stereo earphones that provide visual and auditory cues that depict being a "Virtual Vietnam."

Finally, a discussion about the treatment of PTSD would not be complete without mentioning eye movement desensitization and reprocessing (EMDR) (Shapiro, 2002). Although, debate about the efficacy of EMDR remains controversial, it is another treatment option that may offer hope to persons with PTSD.

Summary

PTSD is potentially disabling anxiety disorder that may follow exposure to an overwhelming traumatic or life threatening stressor. PTSD symptoms vary, but often emerge within 3 months of the trauma, and may resolve in 6 months or become chronic. Clinicians must identify vulnerable populations and high risk factors associated with PTSD and collaborate with the client and family to develop and implement an individualized plan of care.

There is mounting empirical evidence that integrated mental health care, involving pharmacological and CBT offer promise and relief to persons with PTSD. Specialized educational preparation and clinical expertise are necessary to facilitate emotional and cognitive reprocessing. This chapter has offered some salient points about the treatment of PTSD.

Suggested Reading

American Psychiatric Association (2000). *Diagnostic and statistical manual of mental disorders, 4th edition, Text Revision.* Washington, DC.

Bremner, JD; Vythilingam, M; Vermetten, E; Southwick, SM; McGlashan, T; Nazeer, A; Khan, S; Vaccarino, LV; Soufer, R; Garg, PK; Ng, CK; Staib, LH; Duncan, JS; & Charney, DS (2003). MRI and PET study of defitis in hippocampal structure and function in women with childhood sexual abuse and posttraumatic stress disorder. *American Journal of Psychiatry, 160,* 924–932.

Bryant, RA; Moulds, ML; & Nixon, RV (2003). Cognitive behavior therapy for acute stress disorder: A four-year follow-up study. *Behavior Research Therapy, 41,* 489–494.

LeDoux, J (1998). Fear and the brain: Where have we been, and where are we going? *Biological Psychiatry, 44,* 1229–1238.

Lee, GK; Beaton, RD; & Ensign, J (2003). Eye movement desensitization and reprocessing. A brief and effective treatment for stress. *Journal of Psychosocial Nursing and Mental Health Services, 41*, 22–31.

McCauley, J; Kern, DE; Kolodner, K; Dill, L; Schroeder, AF; DeChant, HK; Ryden, J; Derogatis, LR; & Bass, EG (1997). Clinical characteristics of women with a history of childhood abuse: Unhealed wounds. JAMA, *277*, 1362–1368.

National Institute of Mental Health (NIMH) *Facts about Post-traumatic stress disorder:* http://www.nimh.nih.gov/anxiety/ptsdfacts.cfm

Pitman, RK; Sanders, KM; Zusman, RM; et al (2002). Pilot study of secondary prevention of posttraumatic stress disorder with propranolol. *Biological Psychiatry, 51*, 189–192.

Rothbaum, BO & Foa, EB (1999). Exposure therapy for PTSD. *PTSD Research Quarterly*, 10, 1–6.

Rothbaum, BO; Hodges, L; Alarcon, R; Ready, D; Sharar, F; Graap, K; Pair, J; Herbert, P; Gotz, D; Wills, B; & Baltzell, D (1999). Virtual reality exposure therapy for PTSD Vietnam veterans: A case study. *Journal of Traumatic Stress, 12*, 263–371.

Saigh, PA & Bremner, JD (eds.). (1999). *Post-traumatic stress disorder: A comprehensive text.* New York: Allyn & Bacon.

Shapiro, F)2002). EMDR and the role of the clinician in psychotherapy evaluation: Towards a more comprehensive integration of science and practice. *Journal of Clinical Psychology, 58*, 1453–1463.

Stein, BD; Jaycox, LH; Katoika, SH; et al (2003). A mental health intervention for schoolchildren exposed to violence: A randomized controlled trial. JAMA, *290*, 603–611.

Stimpson, NJ; Thompson, HV; Weightman, AL; et al (2003). Psychiatric disorders in veterans of the Persian Gulf War of 1991: Systematic review. *British Journal of Psychiatry, 182*, 391–403.

Generalized Anxiety Disorder

6

Introduction

Generalized anxiety disorder (GAD) is a chronic and debilitating anxiety disorder that manifests as unfounded and excessive worrying and tension. Clients with GAD often complain of exaggerated worrying about their health, concerns about their families, job and anticipation of disasters. Because of emotional and physical toll worrying has on the client, physical symptoms are common and include fatigue, muscle tension, sleep and concentration disturbances, irritability and agitation and diaphoresis (sweating). They are "keyed" up most of the time with little reprieve because of excessive worrying for a period of at least 6 months (American Psychiatric Association [APA], 2000). If these symptoms occur during childhood they are diagnosed as overanxious disorder (APA, 2000).

Prevalence and Course

1. Approximately 2.8 percent of adults in this country, about 4 million, has GAD

2. Twice as many women as men are affected by GAD

3. This anxiety disorder has an insidious course and may begin across the life span, but the peak time is between childhood and middle age

4. Fifty percent of GAD cases begin in childhood and adolescence

5. GAD runs a fluctuating course with period of intense symptoms, particularly during stressful periods

6. The global impairment of GAD results in high utilization of health care resources

Causative Factors

1. Comorbidities associated with first-degree relatives with depression, substance-related and other anxiety disorders.

2. Genetic vulnerability or sensitivity theories are extrapolated from family and twin studies that indicate the heritability of GAD

3. Dysregulation in major neurochemistry circuits, including gamma amino-butyric acid (GABA), norepinephrine, serotonin, neuropeptides and glutamate (Jetty, Charney & Goddard, 2001)

4. Irregularities in either the amygdala or hippocampus that interferes with modulation of fear conditioning (Charney & Deutch, 1996).

Evaluation

Clinicians working with clients who present with GAD must provide a supportive and therapeutic environment and convey patience and empathy. They must collaborate with the client and family and establish clear treatment goals for target symptoms and duration of therapy. An extensive discussion of the evaluation process is found in Chapter 2. In addition, to the discussion in that chapter, it is imperative for clinicians to recognize that clients with GAD experience high levels of chronic stress and may present with a number of stress related medical conditions including irritable bowel syndrome, GI disturbances, headaches and hypertension. Furthermore, the high prevalence of other psychiatric condition warrants assessing for depression, other anxiety disorders and substance misuse.

Physical Findings

- Headaches
- Elevated blood pressure
- GI disturbances (e.g., nausea, diarrhea or abdominal distress)
- Dry mouth
- Muscle tension
- Fatigue
- Sleep disturbances
- Diaphoresis
- Trembling and shakiness
- Hot flashes

Mental Status Examination

- Excessive and unfounded anxiety and worrying
- Depressed or sad mood

- Concentration difficulties
- Agitation and irritability
- Preoccupations
- Suicidal ideations
- Sense of helplessness and hopelessness
- Apprehension
- Restlessness

Table VII: Major Symptoms of Generalized Anxiety Disorder

A. Excessive anxiety and worrying occurring more days than not for at least 6 months

B. A lack of control over the worry

C. The anxiety and worry are associated with 3 or more of the following:

- Restlessness or feeling "keyed up"
- Easily fatigued
- Concentration disturbances
- Irritability
- Muscle tension
- Sleep disturbances

(APA, 2000)

Treatment Considerations

The treatment of GAD is similar to all anxiety disorders that consist of integrated models of care using pharmacological and cognitive behavioral therapy (CBT) and other psychosocial interventions.

Pharmacological Interventions

Pharmacological options for the treatment of GAD must focus on target symptoms and be prescribed at the lowest effective dose necessary to minimize side effects. SSRIs, novel antidepressants, and anxiolytic (antianxiety) agents have demonstrated efficacy in the treatment of GAD. Specific agents include serotonin-norepinephrine reuptake inhibitors (SNRIs) (venlafaxine XR [Effexor XR]), SSRIs (e.g., paroxetine [Paxil]), benzodiazepines (e.g., alprazolam [Xanax], lorazepam [Ativan])and buspirone [Buspar] and non-benzodiazepine anxiolytic agent (e.g., buspirone [Buspar]). The most common side effects of venlafaxine XR are GI disturbances (e.g., nausea, constipation, anorexia), somnolence, dry mouth, dizziness, diaphoresis, sexual disturbances. [*See* **Appendix A:** Side Effects Associated with SSRIs] (Rickels, Pollack, Sheehan, et al, 2000).

Primary side effects of benzodiazepines include sedation, loss of appetite, ataxia and psychological and physiological addiction. They should be avoided in clients with a history of substance misuse. Major side effects of buspirone include GI problems, dizziness, excitement, nervousness, lightheadedness and headaches. As with other anxiety disorders, treatment that combines pharmacological and CBT is likely to produce positive outcomes in the treatment of GAD.

Cognitive-Behavioral Therapy (CBT) and other Psychosocial Interventions

The most extensively researched psychotherapy in GAD is CBT, which several randomized controlled trials indicated to be efficacious in reducing symptoms of GAD (Dugas & Ladouceur, 2000; Ladouceur, Dugas, Freeston, et al, 2000; Oust & Breitholtz, 2000). The long-term efficacy of CBT continues to be studied along with integrated models of care using pharmacological interventions. Combined treatment of CBT and pharmacological interventions have demonstrated improvement and reduced relapse rates than either treatment alone.

Summary

GAD is a very disabling anxiety disorder that has the potential to result high health care consumption, reduced productivity and high mortality costs. Most researchers agree that the costs of GAD may be related to the chronic course of the disorder.

It is imperative for clinicians to collaborate with the client and develop appropriate pharmacological and psychotherapeutic intervention that reduce symptoms and facilitate higher level of functioning.

Suggested Reading

American Psychiatric Association (2000). *Diagnostic and statistical manual of mental disorders, 4th edition, Text Revision*. Washington, DC.

Antai-Otong, D (in press). Contemporary trends in the treatment of generalized anxiety disorder. *Journal of Psychosocial Nursing and Mental Health Services*.

Charney, DS & Deutch, A (1996). A functional neuroanatomy of anxiety and fear: Implications for the pathophysiology and treatment of anxiety disorders. *Critical Review of Neurobiology, 10,* 419–446.

Dugas, MJ & Ladouceur, R (2000). Treatment of GAD: targeting intolerance of uncertainty in two types of worry. *Behavioral Modification, 24,* 635–657.

Jetty, PV; Charney, DS; & Goddard, AW (2001). Neurobiology of generalized anxiety disorder. *Psychiatric Clinics of North America, 24,* 75–97.

Ladouceur, R; Dugas, MJ; Freeston, MH; Leger, E; Gagnon, F; & Thibodeau, N (2000). Efficacy of a cognitive-behavioral treatment for generalized anxiety disorder: Evaluation in a controlled clinical trial. *Journal of Consulting and Clinical Psychology*, 68, 957–965.

Oust, LG & Breitholtz, E (2000). Applied relaxation vs cognitive therapy in the treatment of generalized anxiety disorder. *Behavioral Research Therapy*, 38, 77–790.

Rickels, K; Pollack, MH; Sheehan, DV; & Haskins, JT (2000) Efficacy of extended-release venlafaxine in nondepressed outpatients with generalized anxiety disorder. *American Journal of Psychiatry*, 157, 968–974.

Appendix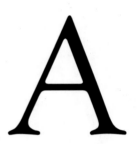

Major Side Effects Associated with SSRIs

- Gastrointestinal disturbances—decreased appetite, diarrhea
- Weight disturbances
- Nervousness, jitteriness, agitation
- Sleep disturbances
- Anxiety
- Tremor
- Discontinuation syndrome with abrupt withdrawal especially with paroxetine
- Diaphoresis (sweating)
- Elevated blood pressure in some clients
- Sexual disturbances
- Hypomania, mania
- Serotonin syndrome

STUDY PACKAGE
CONTINUING EDUCATION CREDIT INFORMATION

Clinicians Update on the Treatment and Management of
Anxiety Disorders

hank you for choosing PESI, LLC as your continuing education provider. Our goal is to ovide you with current, accurate and practical information from the most experienced and nowledgeable speakers and authors.

sted below are the continuing education credit(s) currently available for this self-study package. *Please note, your state licensing board dictates whether self study is an acceptable rm of continuing education. Please refer to your state rules and regulations.*

ocial Workers: PESI, LLC, 1030, is approved as a provider for social work continuing lucation by the Association of Social Work Boards (ASWB), (1-800-225-6880) through the pproved Continuing Education (ACE) program. PESI maintains responsibility for the program. ensed Social Workers should contact their individual state boards to review continuing lucation requirements for licensure renewal. Social Workers will receive 2.0 continuing lucation clock hours for completing this self-study package.

sychologists: PESI, LLC is approved by the American Psychological Association to sponsor ntinuing education for psychologists. PESI, LLC maintains responsibility for these materials and eir content. PESI is offering these self-study materials for 2 hours of continuing education credit.

ounselors: PESI, LLC is recognized by the National Board for Certified Counselors to offer ntinuing education for National Certified Counselors. Provider #: 5896. We adhere to NBCC ntinuing Education Guidelines. This self-study package qualifies for 2.0 contact hours.

ddiction Counselors: PESI, LLC is a Provider approved by NAADAC Approved Education ovider Program. Provider #: 366. This self-study package qualifies for 2.5 contact hours.

ocedures: 1. Read written material.

2. Please complete the post-test/evaluation form and mail to the address on the form. **Your test must be post-marked by the expiration date stamped in the upper right hand corner.**

ur completed test/evaluation will be graded. If you receive a passing score (80% and ove), you will be mailed a certificate of successful completion with earned continuing lucation credits. If you do not pass the post-test, you will be sent a letter indicating areas deficiency, references to the appropriate sections of the tape and manual for review and ur post-test. The post-test must be resubmitted and receive a passing grade before credit n be awarded.

you have any questions, please feel free to contact our customer service department at 300-843-7763.

PESI, LLC

200 SPRING ST., P.O. BOX 1000 • EAU CLAIRE, WI 54702-1000
Product Number: ZHS008425   **CE Release Date:** 07/27/07

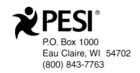

PESI®
P.O. Box 1000
Eau Claire, WI 54702
(800) 843-7763

Clinicians Update on the Treatment
& Management of Anxiety Disorders
Evaluation/Post-test

ZNT008425

This home study package includes CONTINUING EDUCATION FOR ONE PERSON: complete & return this original post/test evaluation form.

ADDITIONAL PERSONS interested in receiving credit may photocopy this form, complete and return with a payment of $15.00 per person CE fee. A certificate of successful completion will be mailed to you.

For office use only
Rcvd. _____
Graded _____
Cert. mld. _____

C.E. Fee: **$15**   Credit card # _____

Exp. Date _____

Signature _____

V-Code* _____ (***MC/VISA/Discover:** last 3-digit # on signature panel on back of card.) (***American Express:** 4-digit # above account # on face of card.)

Mail to: PESI, PO Box 1000, Eau Claire, WI 54702, or
Fax to: PESI (800) 675-5026 (fax all pages)

Name (please print): _____ _____ _____
                          LAST   FIRST   M.I.

Address: _____

City: _____ State: _____ Zip: _____

Daytime Phone: _____

Signature: _____

• Date you completed the PESI Tape/Manual Independent Package: _____

• Actual time (# of hours) taken to complete this offering: _____ hours

PROGRAM OBJECTIVES

How well did we do in achieving our seminar objectives?

	Excellent				Poor
Describe the prevalence of anxiety disorders and their potential burden on individuals and health care systems.	5	4	3	2	1
Review major neurobiological underpinnings of anxiety disorders and implications for treatment.	5	4	3	2	1
Discuss cognitive-behavioral theories associated with anxiety disorders.	5	4	3	2	1
Perform a bio-psychosocial evaluation or assessment that facilitates accurate analysis of client symptoms.	5	4	3	2	1
Differentiate major anxiety disorders and treatment considerations.	5	4	3	2	1
Discuss evidence-based pharmacological agents used in the treatment of diverse anxiety disorders.	5	4	3	2	1
Delineate major psychotherapeutic interventions, such as cognitive behavioral therapies, proven effective in the treatment of anxiety disorders.	5	4	3	2	1
Design an integrated plan of care for the client with an anxiety disorder.	5	4	3	2	1

POST-TEST QUESTIONS

1. Which of the following anxiety disorder(s) has a high comorbidity with major depression?
   a. Generalized anxiety disorder
   b. Panic disorder
   c. Specific phobia
   d. a and b

2. When evaluating clients with anxiety disorders, which of the following is essential in making a differential diagnosis?
   a. Inquiring about caffeine intake.
   b. Asking about substance abuse/dependence.
   c. Ordering appropriate diagnostic studies.
   d. All of the above.

3. Which of the following statements is true about social phobia or social anxiety disorder?
   a. It is very prevalent and often goes unrecognized.
   b. It is seldom found in primary care settings.
   c. It is likely to begin in older adulthood.
   d. It is more difficult to treat than other anxiety disorders.

4. Which of the following is the *most effective* approach for various anxiety disorders?
   a. Benzodiazepines for maintenance treatment.
   b. Novel antidepressant medications for acute treatment.
   c. Cognitive behavioral therapy and antidepressants, and benzodiazepines.
   d. Cognitive behavioral therapy.

5. Mr. Murray, a 45 year old accountant, is seen in the emergency room complaining of chest pain, shortness of breath, fears of dying and going "crazy," and lightheadedness. His physical examination is negative for medical conditions. Which of the following depicts Mr. Murray's symptoms?
   a. Generalized anxiety disorder
   b. Panic disorder
   c. Post Traumatic Stress Disorder (PTSD)
   d. Specific phobia

6. Which of the following medications is likely to reduce Mr. Murray's present symptoms?
   a. Buspirone (Buspar)
   b. Clonazepam (Klonopin)
   c. Fluoxetine (Prozac)
   d. Paroxetine (Paxil)

7. Cognitive behavioral therapy (CBT) is useful in the treatment of various anxiety disorders. Based on the theory of CBT which of the following is the principle aim of treatment?
   a. Enable the client to manage anxiety symptoms more effectively.
   b. Reduce feelings of helplessness or powerlessness.
   c. Work as an adjunct to pharmacological interventions.
   d. All of the above.

**Thank you for your comments.
We strive for excellence and we value your opinion.**

Professional Resources Available from PESI

Resources for Mental Health Professionals

Addiction, Progression & Recovery, by Dale Kesten, LCSW, LADC

Assessing and Treating Trauma and PTSD, by Linda Schupp, Ph.D

Borderline Personality Disorder—Struggling, Understanding, Succeeding, by Colleen E. Warner, Psy.D

Case Management Handbook for Clinicians, by Rand L. Kannenberg, MA

Clinicians Update on the Treatment and Management of Anxiety Disorders, by Deborah Antai-Otong, MS, RN, CNS, NP, CS, FAAN

Collaborative Healing: A Shorter Therapy Approach for Survivors of Sexual Abuse, by Mark Hirschfeld, LCSW-C, BCD & Jill B. Cody, MA

Delirium–The Mistaken Confusion, by Debra Cason-McNeeley, MSN, RNCS

Depression and Other Mood Disorders, by Deborah Antai-Otong, MS, RN, CNS, NP, CS, FAAN

Effective Strategies for Helping Couples and Families, by John S. Carpenter

Grief: Normal, Complicated, Traumatic, by Linda Schupp, Ph.D

Psychiatric Emergencies, by Deborah Antai-Otong, MS, RN, CNS, NP, CS, FAAN

Sociotherapy for Sociopaths: Resocial Group, by Rand L. Kannenberg, MA

Resources for Nurses & Other Healthcare Professionals

Heart and Lung Sounds Reference Library (Audio CD), by Diane Wrigley, PA-C

Infection Control and Emerging Infectious Diseases, by William Barry Inman

Legal and Ethical Standards for Nurses, by Sheryl Feutz-Harter

Managing Urinary Incontinence (Audio CD), by Carol Ann White, RN, MS, ANPC, GNPC

Mechanisms and Treatment of Disease: Pathophysiology—A Plain English Approach, by Mikel A. Rothenberg, MD

Oral Medication and Insulin Therapies: A Practical Guide for Reaching Diabetes Target Goals, by Charlene Freeman

Subclinical Signs of Impending Doom (Audio CD), by Carol Whiteside, RN, PhD(c)

Understanding X-Rays–A Plain English Approach, by Mikel A. Rothenberg

To order these or other PESI products or to receive information about our national seminars, please call 800-843-7763

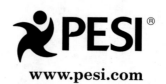

www.pesi.com